HOW TO ELIMINATE ACNE FOREVER

COMBAT PIMPLES ON THE FACE IN WOMEN AND MEN, DEFINITIVE JUVENILE TREATMENT

HOME REMEDIES TO PREVENT ACNE AND BLACKHEADS

Jessy M. Brown

Table of Contents

Introduction

You have seen countless evening infomercials that promise immediate cure to your acne problems... before and after photos showing shocking results from those who have taken a leap of faith and handed over their credit card number for another attempt to successfully remove the acne from their lives forever....

The problem is that you have tried all those remedies, instant "cures", solutions, treatments and creams. You've been through ringer spending a small fortune on acne medications alone to find yourself confused and frustrated as to why you haven't been able to experience the same results everyone claims to have.

As someone who has suffered from

severe acne for many years, I am happy to inform you that your constant suffering from acne is about to end, forever.

Through years of trial and error, trials, spending thousands of dollars on treatments, and dealing with advanced health experts and experienced dermatologists, I finally conquered my acne demon.

Although it took many years before I discovered that most of the highly promoted treatments and solutions for those of us who suffer from acne can intensify our acne and cause excessive breakouts, it took me even longer before I reached the point in my life when acne was a thing of the past.

Had I known about the strategies you are about to discover, I would have saved myself years of pain and anxiety.

   High school could have been a bombshell and I could have had the courage to invite that girl to prom. In college, I may have joined the football team, and at age 20, job interviews and profile photos may have been much easier to handle.

Acne almost destroyed my life, and after so many years of being a pharmaceutical guinea pig, and having spent more money than I care to admit on solutions and treatments only to end up right where I started, I decided to tear down the walls of secrecy and crush the lies and myths that plague and persecute anyone who is dealing with acne.

I spent months compiling my entire strategy within this ebook, so that people just like you, who are suffering unnecessarily, can begin to improve the quality of their life by putting a permanent end to their acne nightmare.

And that's exactly what it is, isn't it? A nightmare.

Acne takes an incredible toll on our minds and bodies. Not only is it a cosmetic problem, acne is often responsible for sleepless nights, incredible pain and loss of confidence and self-esteem.

Even the largest social butterfly will eventually hide under the power of acne in the back of the room, avoiding being photographed, constantly afraid of being noticed.

It all ends today. While these home treatments and remedies take some time to work, if you take action and follow the information contained in this book, you will be able to control and **finally eliminate the acne from your life, permanently**.

So, have a drink, turn off the TV and prepare for an eye-opening adventure in the different methods of regaining control of your life and defeating your acne, once and for all.

Let's get started!

The Truth About Acne

There are so many misconceptions about exactly what causes acne and why certain people suffer from it, while others live a life without blemishes, never having to experience the pain of excessive acne.

With these myths and ridiculous notions comes another series of problems. People who suffer from acne are so desperate to get rid of it that they try all kinds of different approaches, from modifying their diet, to excess tanning believing that it will permanently minimize acne.

These methods can end up being detrimental to your attempts to control your acne, and in many cases can intensify your acne and make it worse. In some cases, these "instant healing remedies" can end up causing permanent scarring.

So what's acne really about?

To begin with, no matter what you've heard, acne is not a threat to life and no one has ever died of acne itself. In clinical terms, acne is described as caused by a hormonal imbalance, clinically coined as"chronic inflammation" or"systemic inflammation.

With chronic inflammation, the main culprit is poor digestion, accompanied by a poor diet.

Another primary cause of acne is when your body's pores become clogged, typically your face, neck, upper body, back and even chest.

When it comes to different types of acne, there are five individual categories based on severity and skin damage caused by acne, including:

- **Comedones**
- **Papule**
- **Pustular Nodule**
- **Cyst**

Acne symptoms, such as blackheads and whiteheads, belong to the comedo category, and cysts are classified as belonging to the nodules category.

Another word for acne is "Acne Vulgaris", a form of acne, which commonly occurs during puberty.

It mainly affects the back, face and chest. Acne vulgaris affects both boys and adolescent girls. Nearly 30-40% of adolescent boys are affected between the ages of 18 and 19. Girls are usually affected between the ages of 16 and 18.

This is how acne is characterized by certain groups that can determine the severity of your acne:

Black heads

You will suffer from blackheads when your pores are partially blocked, allowing some bacteria, dead skin cells and sebum to escape and drain to the surface of your skin.

   The dark color that comes with blackheads is not dirt, so constantly washing your face will not prevent blackheads from appearing. Blackheads are firmer and often take a few days to a week to disappear.

White heads

You will see that white heads appear when a pore is completely blocked, the opposite of a black head.

With white heads, they tend to last only a short period of time and are the result of sebum, bacteria and dead skin cells being trapped under the surface of the skin.

Papules:

 are red, painful bumps that are swollen and do not contain a head.

Pustules

A pustula is what we commonly call a "grain". They are very similar to a white head but are always inflamed and contain a white or yellow center.

Nodules: The nodules

They are larger spots that can last for months and be difficult to treat because of how painful they can be. Nodules are hardened lumps under the surface of the skin. With nodules, scarring is fairly common.

If you think you have nodules, please do not squeeze them, as doing so may cause severe trauma to your skin, spread of the nodules, and prolonged life.

Do not try to treat the nodules on your own, instead, make an appointment with your dermatologist for help, as nodules are quite difficult to control with over-the-counter medications or home remedies.

Cysts

Like a nodule, cysts can be large and hard; in fact, some cysts feel like round balls inside the skin.

They are also very painful and filled with fluid. **Do not squeeze or try to break a cyst**, as it can push bacteria and infection deeper into your skin.

Apart from the common forms of acne that many of us have experienced from time to time throughout our lives, there are four types of acne that are considered more serious and should be treated by a doctor.

Acne Conglobata

This is the most severe form of acne, usually characterized by the large appearance of numerous nodules, often connected, interconnected and containing a large number of blackheads. Because these lesions can become ulcerated, they can cause disfigurement and severe scarring on the surface of the skin.

Conglobata is usually found on the face, back, chest, upper arms, and thighs.

Acne conglobata usually affects people between the ages of 18 and 30 and is more common in men.

It should also be noted that acne Conglobata could remain active for many years, remaining inactive until something happens that causes acne to resurface. The cause of acne conglobata is unknown at this time.

Acne Fulminants

This type of severe acne is actually an abrupt onset of acne conglobata that typically afflicts young men.

The symptoms of severe, often ulcerative, *nodulocystic* acne are easily apparent. As in normal cases of congenital acne, the lesions cover large portions of the extremities and facial region, including disfiguring scars that may eventually develop.

However, what makes fulminant acne unique is that it also includes symptoms of fever, joint pain, especially in the knees and hips, and varying degrees of weight loss depending on the individual.

Folliculitis Gram negative

Gram-negative folliculitis is a form of extreme acne caused by inflammation of the follicles caused by a bacterial infection:

This condition is characterized by **pustules and cysts.**

It has been determined in some cases that its development is caused by a complication resulting from a long-term antibiotic treatment of acne vulgaris.

The reason why this form of acne is called "gram-negative" is related to the fact that gram is a type of blue stain used for laboratory testing of microscopic organisms. Bacteria that do not stain blue are called "gram-negative.

Like other forms of extreme or severe

acne, gram-negative folliculitis is a rare condition, and we do not know if it is more common in men or women, as it has been documented in both.

Pioderma facial

This type of severe acne affects only women, usually between the ages of 20 and 40.

It is characterized by large painful nodules, pustules, and sores that can leave scars.

With abrupt formation, facial pyoderma can appear on the skin of a woman who has never had acne before.

Generally, this type of extreme acne is

limited to the face, and although it does not last more than a year, it can cause a great deal of damage in a very short time.

Keloid is a scar-like acne that may be present in both men and women, however it is more common among men.

Keloid commonly affects the neck area. When swollen papules and pustules become larger cysts and nodules, the skin becomes very oily, causing atrophic and keloid scars on the neck, shoulders, and upper back.

Other types of acne include:

- Acne Rosacea - Most common in the elderly and characterized by red rashes on the chin, nose, cheek and forehead.

- Acne Conglobata - This is a highly inflammatory disease with comedones, nodules, abscesses and draining sinus ducts.

- Acne Fulminans - is a severe form of skin disease, acne, which can occur after an unsuccessful treatment for another form of acne such as acne conglobata.

Acne usually occurs during a person's adolescence, however, adults are not immune to acne, and many of us who don't treat it can end up suffering it all our lives.

Dissected Acne: The Causes

Despite extensive research on the causes of acne and why certain people suffer constantly, while others never experience a single acne attack, it has never been scientifically proven as to the exact cause of acne.

However, there are contributing factors often associated with those who have acne and those who do not, including:

Puberty

Teenagers and pimples always seem to go hand in hand, and it is a time in our lives that even those of us who have never suffered from acne before (or after) experienced the symptoms of the outbreaks.

In fact, studies have revealed that more than 94% of the total population between the ages of 12 and 24 have suffered from acne at one time or another.

The reason acne is so common among teenagers is based on the hormone, androgens, which begin to work as we approach puberty.

Androgens can cause hair follicles and skin pores to enlarge and become extremely oily, and when oil mixes with skin cells, it can cause our pores to become blocked, resulting in temporary outbreaks of acne.

Your hormones

Hormones seem to play an important role in the cause of acne, and have been consistently linked to the cause of severe acne in both adolescents and adults.

It's a family thing.

It has been said that although acne is not directly hereditary, if your parents suffered from severe acne, you are much more prone to acne yourself. Scientists are still studying the links between children with acne and parents and there is no concrete evidence of a direct connection available at this time.

Your recipes

Depending on the type of medication you are taking, certain prescription medications are known to cause an increase in acne, especially antidepressants and anti-anxiety medications, as well as specific types of steroids, barbiturates, and lithium.

If you are taking any medication and think it is causing your acne to get worse, contact your doctor and discuss alternative options based on the prescription you can take to prevent your acne from getting worse.

Do NOT stop taking your medicine until you talk to your family doctor.

Our environment

If you have been exposed to chemicals in your workplace, or even at home with scented cleaners, air fresheners or detergents, you may find that your current acne may become temporarily irritated.

Case studies have also been done where people with no history of acne began experiencing extreme breakouts after

being subjected to continuous chemical
cleaners, especially when they are cleaned
without gloved hands.

"Acne "Natural Remedies

Natural, holistic or home remedies can be an inexpensive way to fight acne.

Natural and herbal remedies are derived from the life of living plants. If each of you has taken a vitamin supplement, you may have noticed the taste just before swallowing it, it tastes like ground plants, leaves, etc., that's because it is. There are no chemicals involved.

Natural herbal remedies do not alter hormonal balance, change chemical levels in the brain, or deceive the body.

Why is that? Because herbs contain certain properties they are intended to regulate the body's functions to promote healing and health.

   They are not synthetic or man-made, they are simply from the earth and they are here to help us with the problems we face. Herbal supplements are a healthy alternative to prescription drugs.

   Some of the natural remedies are listed below.

➤ Beverages rich in antioxidants and vitamin C and/or E can help refresh and rejuvenate the skin.

➤ Foods rich in vitamin E can decrease acne-related scars.

➢ *Tea tree oil is a popular home remedy for acne. It is an essential oil that is diluted and applied topically over acne lesions. Because tea tree oil can kill bacteria, it is believed that the application of topical tea tree oil to acne lesions kills the bacteria that cause acne.

In addition, there are certain herbs that can be digested that can alleviate chronic inflammatory problems especially related to the skin, such as acne.

These herbs include burdock, blades, red clover, fig tree, pica root, echinacea and blue flag. A great combination is the blue flag, burdock, yellow dock and echinacea. These can be mixed together and infused with hot water to make a tea.

Drink a cup of this three times a day.

You can put some honey on it so it tastes better.

When researching over-the-counter options, always focus on medications or ointments containing **5 percent benzoyl peroxide**.

Apply this to problem areas before bedtime, every day.

Benzoyl helps with open sores and pimples, in addition to unblocking blackheads and eliminating bacteria that commonly inhabit skin pores. You should only need a small amount, only one fingertip measurement will do.

Benzoyl peroxide effectively kills bacteria, dries the skin and promotes renewed growth of new cells.

You can buy lower doses without a prescription, however, stronger forms will require a prescription.

"Here are some of my favorite home remedies to instantly treat acne:"

Hot and cold compresses

This is one of the most popular home remedies and very easy to try. All you have to do is wet a towel and press it against the area of your body that has acne, whether it's your face, chest or back.

This will reduce swelling and instantly eliminate clogged pores, which is one of the main culprits in causing acne.

Natural Fruit Juice

A simple but effective strategy is to use natural fruit juices as a way to relieve the presence of external cysts and painful blackheads.

You use these juices as a topical application, stirring a little cucumber or citrus juice with a little almond oil.

Once mixed, apply to the entire area where acne exists and leave on for 15 minutes. Rinse with warm water and pat dry.

Almond oil and other natural substances like it, are easy remedies that will help eliminate acne if applied regularly.

Do this 2-3 times a week.

You can also replace cucumber juice with apricot juice or lemon juice, as long as they are natural and contain no sweeteners or sugars.

Fenugreeks Leaf Remedy

Instead of curing acne, fenugreek leaves help prevent acne from coming back once you have it under control. Simply grind the leaves in a small bowl and add water to form a paste.

Apply this to your face, like a mask, and leave it on overnight. Be sure to use an old pillowcase, as it may leave light stains.

Honey mask

Honey contains natural antibacterial qualities and is often used as a mask in spas and home treatments. These masks are cheap and can be purchased at your local pharmacy.

Apply the mask once or twice a week and enjoy the results. It works exceptionally well!

White Vinegar Treatment

Once again, this is a topical treatment that works wonders. With a cotton ball, soak in white vinegar and apply to the infected area, leaving it to act for 5 to 15 minutes.

Rinse with cold water. If the vinegar seems too strong, dilute with 1/3 cup water and apply.

Oatmeal Mask

Simply cook a small amount of oatmeal and apply it to your face. Allow this mixture to set on your face for 15 minutes before rinsing.

Oats act as a natural exfoliant, providing instant relief. Try to integrate this method at least twice a week, as it takes very little time and effort and will produce great results.

Yeast solution

Mix 1 tablespoon of dry or fresh yeast with 2 tablespoons of lemon juice; apply to face, wait for it to harden (try not to move), peel or wash with lukewarm water.

Laurel Remedy

Grind bay leaves and blanch in warm water, cool and apply to face. Rinse after ten minutes.

Lettuce solution

Saturate clean, rinsed lettuce leaves in water. Rinse your face with water.

Tea Bag Cure

Mix 2-3 tea bags with a little basil and cook in boiling water for 10-20 minutes. Then apply over the acne with a clean cotton ball.

The home remedies listed above are those that have been used successfully over the years.

Personally, I have found the honey mask to do wonders, and the oatmeal mask formula has helped me keep my acne under control without the need for expensive third party treatments.

Acne Treatment

Since skin conditions differ in so many ways (oily, normal, dry or mixed skin) there is no such thing as a one-size-fits-all acne cure.

Recently, the FDA has approved the use of a gel called Epiduo for acne patients over the age of 12.

Epiduo is a combination of two acne treatments that have been tested over time. 2.5% benzoyl peroxide and 0.1% Adapalene in Epiduo are sold generically and are known as Differin.

The manufacturers of Epiduo, Galderma, had stated in a recent press release that the Epiduo gel has been able to combine the two for the first time and that it would come on the market in early 2009.

Several other over-the-counter medications such as Stri-dex, Clearsil, Clearstick and Oxy Night Watch contain a key ingredient to fight acne: salicylic acid.

If the acne is very severe and a cyst has formed that makes other medications immune, then a potent retinoid called isotretinoin can be used orally.

Oral antibiotics have also been commonly used to keep acne breakouts at bay. Antibiotics help reduce inflammation with high initial doses, which are then gradually reduced. But if the acne becomes resistant to the antibiotic over time, it cannot be controlled.

In the United States, many broad-spectrum antibiotics have been used for the purpose of treating acne.

A visit to a dermatologist for a detailed examination is the best way to find out which treatment will work for you.

Your dermatologist will be able to determine the best treatment for you depending on your acne condition as well as your personal skin type.

Scandalous (but effective) home remedies

If you are willing to walk on the wild side and risk the strange, inquisitive looks of friends and family members who might catch you on the spot, here are my favorite home acne remedies ;)

NOTE: All of these remedies are completely safe.

Toothpaste solution

When I first heard about this home remedy, I'm going to be honest, I thought there was no way this was going to work. However, with nothing to lose, I decided to try and was very happy.

Not only does it work exceptionally well,

but it also takes only a few seconds to do so.

All you need is a touch of your favorite toothpaste.

Apply a small amount to your acne blemishes, sores and pimples and let it dry overnight. (Be sure to use an old pillowcase).

You can also replace toothpaste with baking soda and water.

Rinse in the morning and that's it. Do this 2-3 times a week during painful flare-ups

Aspirin Mask

Dermatologists have approved aspirin as

a way to develop a mask to help fight acne. This is a safe and effective method and not only has the potential to relieve acne, but can also help minimize existing scars!

Here's how to create your aspirin mask:

Supplies:

Honey

Uncoated aspirin (any brand)

Neutrogena Healthy Skin Anti-Wrinkle Cream

Alcohol-Free Skin Tonic

Recipe:

- 1) Take four tablets of aspirin and place them in a small

container.

2) Spray water on the aspirin. Do NOT use too much water, or the aspirin will dissolve, just sprinkle a few drops to loosen it. Using your fingers, rub the water and aspirin together to mix well and separate the tablets.

   -   The texture of the mixture must be very granular.

3) Now, add two teaspoons of honey to your mixture. Mix the formula well so that aspirin, water and honey mix well.

4) Apply the mixture to your face making sure it does not get into your eyes. Once your face is completely covered with the aspirin mask, leave it on for ten minutes.

-    Don't touch it or scrub it once it's on your face. After ten minutes, rinse your face formula with cold water, which rubs the aspirin beads all over your face (exfoliating your skin).

5) Then, after washing your skin, use the tonic to dry your face, smoothing it everywhere. This will also remove excess formula and leave your face looking like new.

6) And finally, use the moisturizer you bought as a finishing touch to polish your face and replace moisture. Your moisturizer should contain retinol, which will tighten your face and reduce the appearance of wrinkles and lines.

Repeat 2-3 times per week.

Ice, Ice Baby

Another easy home remedy that worked wonders every time I used this method during extreme outbreaks. All you have to do is apply a cold, compact ice pack (or a broken ice pack) to your face every night before going to bed.

A wet towel will also work well, as it will reduce swelling and help eliminate clogged pores that cause outbreaks.

Milk of magnesia (three-part process)

This is a great household cleaner that is absolutely safe to use. Simply apply to the infected area and leave on for 10-15 minutes before rinsing.

Then, dissolve one teaspoon of Epsom salt (magnesium sulfate) in 3/4 of hot water.

Apply to the infected area with a clean cloth (avoid cotton balls as they may stick to the skin and clog pores). Leave on for 20 minutes before rinsing with cold water.

Finally, the third part consists of creating a homemade toner. Simply add 3 drops of benzoin or peroxide oil to a cup of cold water.

Wash your face with this solution and rinse.

This is an antibacterial remedy, and it works very well, so try it!

Sandalwood powder

All you need for this remedy is a teaspoon of sandalwood powder and a teaspoon of tumeric.

Mix this with a small amount of white milk (any kind). Distribute it in the infected areas and let it act for 15 to 25 minutes. Rinse with warm water and pat dry.

This may take a couple of sessions to get started but produces incredible results. Again, it's totally safe to do as many times as you want.

The oil strategy

This is one of the most effective methods I have tried, and it was a regular routine during extreme acne attacks and breakouts.

All you need for this acne-free recipe is a small bottle of castor oil, and a small bottle of extra virgin olive oil or jojoba oil, which works just as well. Virgin oil will provide moisture to your skin and also eliminate any bacteria that may be trapped under the surface of your skin.

In addition, virgin oil also fortifies the skin with its natural antioxidants.

Create a mixture of 1/2 olive oil and 1/2 castor oil, also mixed. You can experiment with other portions later, but when you start it is always recommended to start with a mixture equal to half and half.

Once mixed, gently massage into all affected areas of the body (can be used anywhere, including the face, neck, upper body and back). Once smoothed in all infected areas, place a warm towel or cloth over the area for 10-15 minutes.

What this does is naturally vaporize your face, allowing your pores to breathe and open, releasing toxins from beneath the surface of your skin.

Leave the solution in your body with the compact serving as a sealer for 10-15 minutes. Then massage the oils back into your skin before rinsing it with cold water (not hot, as the cold will tighten your skin and close your pores).

If you decide to use olive oil, be sure to buy extra virgin olive oil, not normal olive oil, as it will contain fewer impurities. You can also replace olive oil with jojoba oil, which works very well.

One vitamin a day, keeps acne at bay

Taking a multivitamin every day can help control acne by making sure your skin is properly nourished and that your body is not producing an abundance of sebum (which is responsible for clogged pores).

Another useful tip is to add chromium to your diet, a supplement focused on curing skin infections.

Acne Scar Removal

If you've been left with excessive scars caused by acne, there are things you can do to minimize and eliminate the scars.

One of these options is called laser resurfacing, which is performed within a hospital or medical center by a physician or dermatologist, and is a corrective surgical method that quickly eliminates the appearance of scars. With this technique, the top layer of skin is removed, revealing a clean, fresh and scarless layer.

This is similar to laser eye surgery, in which a thin layer of damaged tissue is removed to expose a new, intact layer, instantly correcting and removing any scarring or damage.

The only disadvantage of this procedure is the costs involved. Re-surface can be very expensive, however, it is a safe method of permanently removing scars caused by extreme acne.

For deep acne scars, there is a procedure called a punch graft. This is where good, healthy skin is removed from other parts of the body and used to replace scarred skin by grafting.

If you are interested in learning more about these methods, contact your local dermatologist for a free consultation.

Laser resurfacing is the only definitive solution for removing permanent scars, however, there are also home remedies that fade scars, but do not completely remove them.

One of these treatments is completed by rubbing vitamin E into the scar area. You can buy vitamin E in liquid form, or as a capsule that you can cut out and remove the vitamin to rub on your scarred areas.

You can also try rubbing virgin olive oil on your scars regularly, which has been said to help reduce the appearance of scars.

Treating Acne with Medicines

Acne medications can be topical or systemic.

Topical medications should be applied to the skin where they are taken as systemic medications. The main goal of medications is to eliminate acne from the roots by healing the factors that lead to the formation of acne.

These are some of the medicines used to treat acne.

Oral antibiotics are often used to cure acne. It is usually administered to people who suffer from acne consistently.

However, the bacteria that cause acne may soon become impermeable to antibiotics and thus refuse to treat acne. Doctors will then usually prescribe a different round of antibiotics to help the cause. The most common types of antibiotics used are erythromycin and tertracycline and their derivatives.

However, erythromycin causes discomfort in the gastrointestinal tract and tetracycline and its derivatives are not suitable for pregnant women and children under the age of eight. The components of these antibiotics cure the pustule or swelling by drying it internally.

Topical retinoids are another set of medications used to treat acne. They are derived from vitamin A and may prevent pores from closing. In doing so, they don't really allow acne to form.

They include gels or creams such as adapalene, tazarotene and tretinoin. Topical retinoids may cause rashes and other irritations. They can cause sunburn because your skin will become more vulnerable to UV rays when using this product.

You would need to use sunscreen if these creams are applied. It is important to contact your skin specialist before opting for these medications.

Corticosteroid injections are given to acne patients only when the acne has swollen to the point of bursting. Thus the swelling decreases and the acne dries at a faster rate.

For cystic acne and severe cases of acne, isoretinoin is used. This is only for extreme cases and to cure intricate acne problems.

Oral contraceptives are effective medications to cure acne, but they also have their limitations. They are not intended for women who smoke, women over the age of 35, or women who suffer from problems related to blood clotting.

Oral contraceptives decrease excess

secretion from the glands and thus regulate hormones to control acne.

Tropical antimicrobials are used to treat moderate acne problems. These drugs attack bacterial colonies.

These medications can be taken individually or in combination with others that treat certain causes of acne formation. They include azelaic acid, benzoyl peroxide, clindamycin, erythromycin and sodium sulfatamide. Where azelaic acid and clindamycin decrease bacterial growth, benzoyl peroxide kills bacteria to treat acne.

A mixture of erythromycin with benzoyl peroxide is extremely effective in the treatment of acne. However, these drugs have certain adverse effects.

Acne and Hormonal Balance Treatment

Hormones play a very important role in the formation of acne. The male hormone, androgen, as well as the female hormone, estrogen, contribute to the formation of acne.

These hormones are released during puberty and also during menstruation and pregnancy. This is why a higher percentage of women compared to men suffer from acne.

A proper hormonal balance can be achieved by several methods. These include healthy eating habits, getting rid of stress, drinking plenty of water, and also exercising regularly.

These excess harmful toxins, as well as hormones, need to be excreted from your system. This is usually done by the kidneys and liver.

However, what you need to understand is that these organs cannot function effectively if you have an unhealthy diet. You must eat a well-balanced meal so that your body receives all the necessary nutrients and can work efficiently.

Too much of any constituent will eventually lead to the loss of another and damage your body's system. This will damage your skin.

Natural treatments include the use of antioxidants that balance hormones and also cleanse the blood so that it is free of harmful toxins.

Also, try to drink plenty of water and stay away from coffee can keep acne breakouts at bay. Avoid stress and anxiety, exercise regularly, and stay away from fatty foods. All of these measures tend to restrict the release of excess hormones and prevent the formation of acne.

Corticosteroids are effective in reducing blemishes. But too much of this type of medication can also be harmful - that's why you should always consult your doctor before deciding to take it.

The best way to balance hormones is through natural processes. They guarantee great results and carry with them, with no risk of side effects.

The Best Acne Nutritional Diet

For those who have acne, it is a very good idea to have a diet that contains an abundance of fresh fruits and vegetables. Also, be sure to drink plenty of water regularly to keep your system clean and toxins consistently removed from your system. Eight or ten glasses a day will suffice.

Another good idea is to focus on incorporating a diet rich in antioxidants and fiber.

These are dietary ingredients that will keep your skin healthy and fit and allow you to look good and feel good.

Another thing that is considered very good at fighting acne is protein. Vitamin A is also considered by health experts as a great weapon against acne.

Oregon Grap and Echinacea

These are two herbs that are exceptional for stimulating your body's immune system and will also help minimize the bacteria that are known to trigger or cause acne breakouts.

Educate Yourself About Acne

If you think acne only affects teenagers, then think again. Commonly attacks adults on a daily basis. It can be overwhelming to start noticing sprouts of pimples, pimples or pimples all over your face and you may not know what to do first.

Before doing anything else, visit or call your local pharmacist. Licensed pharmacists always know the skin products and will know which products relieve acne and which do not. Most pharmacists are very willing to help. If you don't already know one, try your local WalMart.

While at WalMart, take a look at some of

the natural remedies available and products that have been displayed near the pharmacy. Many natural products claim to completely cure your acne. Any good pharmacy will also have exhibits of various supplements that claim to help alleviate acne.

Learn about the different causes of acne and discover what is causing your own skin to break down. Acne research is long and still ongoing so experts aren't absolutely sure about the precise causes of acne. However, there are some possible causes on which everyone seems to agree.

Medicines

Some medications, such as steroids, barbiturates, and anticonvulsants, are thought to contribute to skin disorders. However, do not stop taking prescription medications before consulting your doctor to see if they could be causing your acne.

Emotional stress

Increasing evidence suggests that stress can contribute to acne and other skin problems. If you are stressed, try to develop an exercise program and follow it regularly. Exercise has been shown to break stress.

Chocolate

Chocolate has not yet been shown to cause acne. Many people insist that eating chocolate will make you get pimples, but no research has shown this theory to be true.

Cosmetics

Because acne is triggered by clogged or

blocked pores, we can safely assume that makeup and other oil-containing cosmetic products will contribute to acne. Even "safe" products (those that are hypoallergenic and oil-free) can contribute to the formation of blackheads or pimples because they cover the skin. Any cosmetic product applied to the skin has the potential to clog pores and interfere with acne treatment.

Rubbing your face often

Acne-prone skin should always be kept clean, but only mild products should be used.

to wash it gently. Many people have the impression that they should rub the skin with strong soaps when they have acne, but this only aggravates and worsens the condition.

Contamination

High humidity and other unnatural environmental conditions (i.e., smog, fog) can promote acne as well as other disorders. If the skin is exposed to moist conditions for a prolonged period of time, swelling (which blocks the pores, thus contributing to acne) occurs.

Eating Habits

Many people notice that certain foods they eat cause their acne to get worse. Your eating habits can certainly contribute to outbreaks and you should consider the products that cause most problems so you can avoid them in the future.

Common culprits of foods believed to worsen acne include fats and dairy products. Diets rich in zinc should be beneficial if you have acne. Taking zinc supplements is an alternative you might consider for acne relief or treatment.

Causes and Best Treatments for Your Acne

No one in the world is immune to acne. It affects people of all walks of life and all age groups. Acne does not show preferential treatment towards men, women, the rich or the poor. Because each person's skin is different, they all have different contributing factors that cause their particular type of acne.

The most important part of your acne treatment is to understand what type of skin you are and the most effective acne treatment to use on it. If you have oily skin, you don't want to use cleansers, moisturizers, or cosmetics that contain oil.

You must buy products that do not

contain oil. On the other hand, if you have dry skin, you won't want to use the fat-free products because your skin might use a little more fat.

Both oily and dry skin need to be hydrated daily. Just because the skin is greasier doesn't mean it doesn't need hydration. There are many good oil-free moisturizers available for use on oily skin. Dry skin has its own specific problems and should be hydrated with a product made especially for dry skin.

Topical skin treatments are designed to prevent pores from clogging while removing excess dirt and grease on the skin's surface, as well as the bacteria that cause acne. There are certain oral medications that will keep your body from making so much oil. Prescription creams and ointments will help keep breakouts dry and even promote rapid cell replacement in those areas of acne-infected skin that need it. There are other medical and natural remedies that help in the treatment of acne.

Before you understand how to develop the right acne skin care treatment for your skin, you should try to understand what is causing acne in the first place.

Acne Causes

Acne has many causes and all of them are not fully understood or corroborated yet. Some of the most common causes are listed below:

✓ Hormones play an important role in the development of acne. Early adolescence brings many hormonal changes to the body, and those changes often cause constant outbreaks of pimples, pustules, and even cysts.   The adult years also bring changes, especially for women. Premenstrual and premenopausal difficulties cause outbreaks in an alarming number of women. Due to the excess oil produced during acne caused by hormones, products that help eliminate and reduce oil will be more useful for this type of acne.

✓ Stress is certainly a common factor in acne development. When the body becomes tense, it releases chemicals and hormones that eventually become toxins and wastes that the body must expel. Some of these waste products are excreted through the skin and contribute to acne.

✓ Some people still believe that chocolate, sugar and other foods can cause acne to form. Most experts deny that food has anything to do with the development of acne, but the issue is still widely debated and researched, so we cannot be absolutely sure that certain foods do not contribute to acne.

✓ Cosmetics and skin care products can also contribute to acne if the products used are not the right skin type. The use of oily products on oily skin can certainly contribute to breakouts, so it is important to choose your personal care products very carefully when deciding which is the best treatment for acne on your skin.

Other factors, such as lifestyle and the

environment, can also affect your skin.
The best thing you can do for your skin is
to learn how to properly care for it, keep it
hydrated, keep it hydrated and try to
eliminate the factors that are causing your
skin to have acne.

5 Simple Guidelines For The Success Of Your Acne Skin Treatment

People with acne consider it an annoying problem, one that frustrates them to the point of hopelessness.

Acne skin treatment takes time once acne has developed, but the truth is, if acne has not already started, then it is fairly easy to prevent its appearance. If it has begun to appear, then after your prescribed acne treatment it should bring positive results in a short period of time.

No matter what your situation, you can have healthy skin if you have some guidelines for proper skin care in mind.

Keep your skin clean

Perhaps the most important part of your daily skin care regimen is keeping it clean. It should be washed twice a day, morning and night, with a mild hypoallergenic cleanser. In addition, you should clean up after any activity that makes you sweat an abnormal amount, such as strenuous activity or exercise.

The most important thing is the type of cleanser you use on your skin. Rubbing your skin with a harsh and abrasive soap will only worsen your acne. If you don't know a good cleanser for your skin type, consult your dermatologist for advice. Once you have washed your skin (gently), rinse and pat dry.

If your hair is oily, like your skin, then it should be shampooed daily because the grease in your hair can easily reach your face and cause problems.

Careful shaving

Shaving is a problem that usually only affects men. The choice of shaver type (electric or safety) depends on which is the easiest and most comfortable to use. When safety razor blades are used, the short blade should be the only one used on acne-prone skin. Before applying the shaving foam, the beard should be softened with soap and water. Shave very carefully and gently to avoid irritating imperfections that may be present.

Keep your hands away from your face.

Manipulating (squeezing or popping) bumps on the face will only cause ugly acne scars to spread or form. Keep your fingers completely away from your acne blemishes or you run the risk of interfering with your acne treatment.

Cosmetics

Check your makeup products to make sure they are hypoallergenic and oil-free. If they do, or if they are old, you should throw them away and buy new products. Be sure to read product labels to make sure they do not contain ingredients that may conflict with your acne treatment. Until your treatment progresses, it may be difficult to use foundation makeup or other liquid makeup products on your skin.

In addition to checking your makeup, you should also look at the shampoo and conditioner you use on your hair. If they contain oil, acne may begin to appear on the forehead. Make sure all hair products are not comedogenic.

Stay out of the sun

Even if you think that tanned skin makes your blemishes look better, be careful not to expose your skin to the sun, especially during the acne skin treatment period. Prolonged exposure to the sun will quickly age your skin and put you at risk for skin cancer.

In addition to the sun's harmful effects on the skin, the acne medication you are using may react negatively when exposed to the sun's rays, making it much more likely to burn with the sun.

5 Facts About Acne Treatment

Just the mention of the word "acne" fills some people with fear. They foresee having to spend long hours caring for their skin by rubbing it, applying expensive creams and avoiding the foods they like to eat the most in order to avoid pimples coming out all over their faces.

The big news is that advances are being made in acne treatment and experts are discovering new ways to prevent and treat this dreaded skin condition. Some of the old wives' tales about acne have proven to be false and new information on how to get clear and beautiful skin is being discovered daily.

Check out these 5 little-known facts

about acne treatment and skin care:

1) Scrub or not scrub?

Although experts once thought it was necessary to rub for clean, pimple-free skin, they now know that rubbing the skin with strong abrasives only serves to irritate and injure it. Because the skin is delicate, it can easily be damaged, leaving it unable to act as a shield against harmful bacteria. Therefore, rubbing the skin with or without abrasives should be avoided.

2) Can the sun beautify my skin?

Although the sun is able to stop bacteria in their tracks, it also damages your skin by drying it and clogging its pores. Prolonged exposure (more than 15 minutes a day) to sunlight will not help you get beautiful skin and should be avoided.

3) Will cold air help clear my skin of acne?

Extremely cold weather damages the skin in the same way as sunlight by drying it out and clogging pores. Cold air should be avoided because it will interfere with any progress you are making toward clearing up your acne outbreaks. The best temperature to maintain a beautiful, clear skin is between 70 and 80 degrees F.

4) Will swimming damage my skin?

Swimming is an excellent choice, both for your fitness level and for your acne-prone skin. Swimming in an indoor pool purified with ozone, with water at a temperature of approximately 75 to 85 degrees Fahrenheit, will refresh your irritated skin, reduce stress and provide great exercise for your entire body.

5) How can I avoid contact with the bacteria that cause acne?

The best way to prevent the acne that causes bacteria and have pimple-free skin is to keep everything around you as clean as possible. Bacteria thrive on bedding, towels and cloths, so you should wash them every time you use them. Some natural products that have been shown to reduce bacteria are vinegar, essential oils

and tea tree oil, all of which can be used
to wash linens and underwear.

Following these 5 steps will help you
fight and effectively control your stubborn
acne because you will learn to change
your bad habits.

Changing your unhealthy habits will lead
to a healthier lifestyle that, in turn, will
lead to beautiful, clear, acne-free skin.

Treating Acne in the "Natural" Way

Acne is a common skin disorder that affects the sebaceous glands of the face, back, and neck. Most people are affected by acne at some point in their lives and suffer with the resulting pimples, blackheads, blackheads and cysts.

The sebaceous glands work to expel excess fat from the skin. Invariably, they will become clogged from time to time and the resulting accumulation of oil can cause acne as well as other skin conditions. Acne vulgaris is the most common condition and mainly affects teenagers.

Many factors contribute to acne vulgaris and include nutritional imbalances, allergens, emotional stress, liver abnormalities, heredity, excessively oily skin, certain medications and hormones.

Another factor contributing to acne is the overabundance of toxins and poisons in the body. The body uses the liver and kidneys to get rid of these dangerous substances. If the body contains more impurities than those organs can effectively handle, the skin takes over by sweating the substances.

All these processes that work at the same time alter the body's natural healing capacity and create various skin conditions, causing the formation of pimples and blackheads.

There are many natural products available that will effectively treat acne. Listed below are several of the best and well-tolerated alternative methods to eliminate the effects of acne.

Note, however, that some of these methods may have to be repeated over the course of 2 to 4 weeks before lasting results are noticed.

➢ Apply white vinegar (distilled and diluted if necessary) to areas of skin affected by acne. Allow it to remain on the skin for up to 10 minutes and then rinse gently with cold water.

➢ Use Echinacea daily to improve immunity.

➢ Take Oregon grape daily to protect against acne-causing bacteria.

➢   Apply lemon juice to areas of the face affected by pimples, blackheads, and other skin conditions. Let juice remain on face for up to 10 minutes, then rinse with cold water. Other citrus juices may be used and diluted if they cause itching sensations. This solution will function as a natural exfoliant by rubbing dead skin tissue.

➢   Use dandelion or red clover daily to remove toxins from the liver.

➢   Use Natures Sunshine's Ayurvedic Skin Detox to remove liver toxins.

➢ Use of vitamin A supplements will help severe acne. Consult your doctor to determine the correct dose because too large amounts can be toxic.

➢ Take zinc supplements to stimulate tissue repair and prevent skin scarring.

➢ Try Alternative Homeopathic Remedies to dry pimples and heal damaged tissues.

➢ Eat a well-balanced diet and take vitamin and mineral supplements to prevent nutritional deficiencies. Keeping your body healthy will promote the natural healing of your tissues.

> Drink plenty of water daily to eliminate toxins and keep the body hydrated.

Common Acne Myths

People still believe in old wives' tales about the causes of acne, even though experts have refuted many of the myths. We will try to reveal the truth about some of those hard myths and reassure you so that you can advance in your search for a clear, acne-free and beautiful skin.

Myth: Only dirty people have acne

Fact: Acne is not caused by poor hygiene, but by hormonal changes that occur inside the body. Sometimes the sebaceous glands (responsible for moisturizing our skin) fill with fat and block nearby follicles. This causes clogged pores, which turn into acne characterized by pimples, blackheads, pustules, and even cysts.

The truth is that rubbing and washing your skin consistently can make your acne problem much worse. Proper skin care routine involves gently washing the skin and patting it dry (without rubbing).

Myth: People with acne aren't eating the right foods.

Reality: Experts now know that there is no connection between the foods you eat and the development of acne.

The myths that chocolate and other fattening foods cause acne are completely wrong. On the other hand, you need to practice proper nutrition for your overall health to be excellent.

Myth: Stress causes acne

Fact: Stress itself does not cause acne, although it can develop as a side effect when taking prescription medications to help you deal with stress. If you take this type of medication and notice symptoms of acne, such as pimples, pimples, or pustules, consult with your doctor to determine if the medication could be contributing to your skin condition. A word of caution: although stress won't cause acne, it can make the condition worse if you already have it.

Myth: Acne is purely cosmetic

Fact: Acne changes your appearance, but it can also pose a threat to your mental health. Severe acne problems, often characterized by cystic nodules and persistent eruptions, can lead to severe acne, causing permanent scarring.

This sometimes affects people

psychologically by altering their self-image. Many people develop self-esteem problems and feel frustrated and depressed.

Myth: Acne is incurable

Fact: Acne can be completely cleared up by using the many products available and finding the right treatment specific to your needs.

Your dermatologist can help you find the best method to treat your acne and will be able to determine what type of acne you have, whether it is acne vulgaris, acne cysticus, acne nodularis, or even rosacea. There are good and effective treatments and medications available (including Accutane, Retin-A, and many others) to help clarify even the most persistent problems. Before you know it, it will reveal to you the beautiful skin you should always have had.

Creative use of makeup to hide acne

You finally took that important step by visiting your dermatologist and starting acne treatment earlier this week! Your skin will soon become clear, beautiful and acne free.

Congratulations! Did you say you had an important meeting to attend tomorrow and needed to have your skin cleared by then? Well, your acne may not clear up as quickly, but there are some tips you can use in order to see your best at your meeting.

Using makeup creatively will allow you to temporarily hide your acne, but you must follow some basic rules. Keep in mind that this is just a cover-up, not a cure.

The Basic Elements Necessary for Your Acne Cover-Up Kit

Your most important tools for covering acne will be concealer, foundation and powder. Buy only branded and trusted products from trusted stores. Choose hypoallergenic and oil-free products that match your skin color.

Read the product labels thoroughly to make sure you are not buying products loaded with oil that will stop the treatment of acne just started on its way. If you decide to try a new brand, try it before you use it by rubbing a little below the jaw line. If your skin is going to react negatively, it will in an hour.

Before the cover-up begins

Before starting the process of covering

acne, gently wash your face and neck with your regular cleanser and then pat dry. Use your new acne medicine below, applying it according to the instructions. Allow to dry completely.

The main event

Now you can start the cover-up process. Apply small amounts of concealer directly onto the red or dark spots on your face and neck that were caused by acne spots. Use a disposable makeup sponge to mix the concealer with your skin.

Do not exaggerate this step because too much corrector will look awful once it dries. Apply very lightly.

Now, apply small amounts of makeup to the skin, mixing it with the sponge. Reapply on areas that seem to need a little more coverage but, again, don't overdo it, because too much makeup will draw attention to your skin with acne scars.

The last step is to apply a very light coat of powder, using a soft make-up brush. Always use oil-free powder with the softest brush you can find to avoid irritating your skin with acne problems. The powder will absorb the shine left by the makeup and will also give your face that "finished" look.

Be sure to get rid of the makeup sponges you used during the cover-up. These will retain the oil from your face and should be discarded to avoid transferring the same oil to your face tomorrow.

Before going to sleep

Always wash your face before going to bed every night. Your skin needs that time to breathe and your acne doesn't need to have a makeup layer, because additional blemishes can result. Reapply acne treatment (as directed).

Acne Scar Repair

Acne, a common skin disorder that people spend millions of dollars trying to cure, usually affects 80% of our youth and 5% of our adult population. Young people, who are the most affected, spend hours agonizing over the devastating effects that acne causes on their skin.

At an early age, they are harassed by social problems and popularity problems. The scars left by your acne battles are detrimental to your ego and your self-esteem. Billions of dollars have been spent on acne research, acne scars, and scar solutions.

There are three classifications of acne scars, Icepick, Boxcar and Rolling. The duration of the scars also causes them to be divided into two other groups, one early and one permanent.

Topical medications work well in early scars, but surgical intervention is often necessary for permanent scarring. Combinations of treatments are sometimes used for both types, depending on their severity. Along with the available topical medications, skin rejuvenation procedures and surgical procedures are also used for more severe scars.

Surgical procedures are expensive treatment options and there are advantages and disadvantages of this type of solution for acne scars. Before using surgery, doctors will evaluate the patient's age, gender, history of medical problems, skin type, and type of scar, among other things.

Sometimes collagen or other injections may be used to elevate the scar to the level of the skin. These injections are called dermal fillers.

The "punching excision" procedure is frequently used by dermatologists when treating scars from ice sticks or freight cars. This procedure involves cutting the skin with a special tool and sewing the edges of the skin together. This forms a new scar that heals with lighter skin. There is also a variation of this procedure, called "puncture excision with skin graft replacement.

It is very similar to the original procedure, except for the skin that is sewn. Instead, it is grafted onto the skin to repair the scar.

The subcutaneous incision is yet another procedure, but it is mainly used in rolling scars. In this procedure, a needle is inserted into the skin and the scar tissue is cut. The skin is bruised a lot during this procedure, but disappears in about a week.

Laser resurfacing burns the top layer of skin, bringing it down to the original level.

When you look at all these procedures used to treat scars, it's obvious that prevention is better than cure.

To prevent scarring, try to avoid the sun, use alpha-hydroxy acids, exercise regularly, and maintain good eating habits. You could save a lot of unnecessary expense and humiliation.

Acne Scar Treatment - Can Acne Scars Be Eliminated?

Scars are indications that the body has repaired itself in one way or another, whether due to injury or infection. Once these events occur, the body's white blood cells accumulate at the site to fight more infections and repair the damage that has occurred.

Once that process is complete, scars often form. This process can be compared to a seam sewn on a torn piece of fabric. The skin (or seam) will never be as smooth as before the damage.

There are different types of acne scars and different degrees of each type. Some people may develop worse scars than others, depending on their individual tendencies.

Types of Acne Scars

There are two different types of acne scars. The first type, depressed scarring, is caused by tissue loss and the second type, keloids, is caused by tissue formation.

1) Depressed scars

This type of scar is caused by the dermis that is attacked by toxins that escape from the skin. Once a cyst breaks, it expels pus, oil, bacteria, and other poisons into the surrounding areas.

White blood cells rush to the site of infection to repair the skin. In the process, valuable collagen is lost, causing recessions or depressions in the skin. The skin above the lesion will develop scars, commonly called ice pick scars. Other types of scars are soft, mascular and fibrous.

2) Keloids

This type of scarring is the result of fibroblasts that the body triggers during the repair process. Once collagen begins to decrease, fibroblasts produce excess collagen, resulting in tissues called keloids. They usually form in the male body and are sometimes called hypertrophic scars.

Acne Scar Treatment

Consult your dermatologist about the best treatment for your individual scars. Be prepared to talk about your feelings about the scars, the cost of treatment, and what you want the end result of treatment to be. Your doctor will need to consult with you regarding the severity and location of the scars, as well as the type of treatments available.

Commonly requested scar treatments include laser, collagen, and dermabrasion. Skin surgery and/or grafting are also considerations if the scars are deep. Keloids are sometimes left alone if the doctor believes that treatment will cause other keloids to form.

In this case, keloids can sometimes be effectively remedied by the use of steroid injections.

Vitamins, minerals, and other acne-eliminating supplements

Many supplements exist that will help accelerate the success of your acne treatment. It is well known that taking certain vitamins, minerals, or other types of supplements will help eliminate skin disorders. We are listing some of the most effective ones to use when fighting acne.

Vitamins

- 50,000 IU of water-soluble vitamin A should be taken just before eating. Do not take more than this amount before getting your doctor's approval because too much vitamin A can be toxic. If you begin to experience unwanted symptoms with this dose, then decrease it to 25,000 IU.

-   500-1000 mg of vitamin B5, or pantothenic acid, should be taken daily.

-   25-150 mg of vitamin B6 should be taken daily (vitamin B6 should be one of the vitamins of a B-complex vitamin).

-   1000 mg of vitamin C buffered should be taken three times daily.

-   400 IU of vitamin E should be taken twice a day and taken before meals.

Minerals

-   One tablet of Calcium Hydroxyapatite Complex should be taken 3 times a day after each meal.

-   200-500 micrograms of Chromium should be taken daily.

-   25-60 mg of Zinc Gluconate should be taken once a day. Never exceed 100 mg unless approved by your doctor. Zinc is by far the most important mineral to take in your quest for acne freedom, as it reduces DHT, the male sex hormone that can cause acne if there is an excessive amount of it in the body.

Oxygen Elements Plus

Oxygen Elements Plus is a nutrient that, with proper use, will add 10-20% more oxygen to your blood. In addition to beneficial oxygen, this product also contains other useful minerals and nutrients.

Acid, waste products and pathogens serve to consume much of the oxygen you receive. The amount left over is the amount your body should use for the rest of your needs. Because you need more oxygen than is available, Oxygen Elements Plus is a great product to help you get it. Your skin needs oxygen to stay clean and free of bacteria. More oxygen can result in clear, acne-free skin.

Other special supplements

There are six special supplements, in addition to Oxygen Elements Plus, that can eliminate acne, as well as improve your level of health and immunity to infections.

- Mineral electrolytes
- Digestive Enzymes
- Lecithin
- Chlorophyll
- Systemic Enzymes
- Flaxseed oil

These supplements should be used according to the instructions on their individual labels.

It is important to stop using any of the supplements mentioned here (especially those with high doses) once your acne is under control.

Once things are back to normal, you should continue any supplemental programs you were originally using. Prolonged use of high-dose supplements can sometimes cause a chemical imbalance in your body and can be harmful to your health.

Conclusion

In order to consistently control and eliminate acne, it is necessary to develop a system that includes a good diet, as well as follow a regimen that incorporates elements to combat acne in your daily life.

Do not deviate from this system until your acne is well under control. It takes time and effort to combat acne, but if you follow the strategies presented in this guide, you will be well on your way to permanently eliminating the acne from your life.

You deserve to look and feel your best. By researching your options, consulting with a skin care specialist and implementing small changes in your diet and environment, you can control acne once and for all.

Now yes, I wish you the best in your results, and remember, everything is practical; theory without action is of no use to you. It brings everything you learn into real life.

A big hug, your friend, Jessy!